A VISIT TO THE LIBRARY

BY
JAMIE STONEBRIDGE

ALSO BY JAMIE STONEBRIDGE

Trip To The Lake
A Day At The Park
A Visit To The Farm
A Day At The Beach
An Autumn Adventure
A Visit To The Library

And more...

amazon.com/author/jamiestonebridge

THANK YOU

It is people like you that keep reading alive. We can all live through books. Reading alone or with others is a wonderful thing.

I hope this book brings you joy and happiness.

You can help other readers discover this book by leaving a review on Amazon.

Special thanks to Thanks to Rachel Horon for her help on this book. She has always been inspired by the libraries in her communities like the Belleville Public Library and Lake County Public Library System. She appreciates the staff, resources, and community activities for patrons of all ages. The joy from volunteering at the library in her youth has been passed down another generation to her own kids.

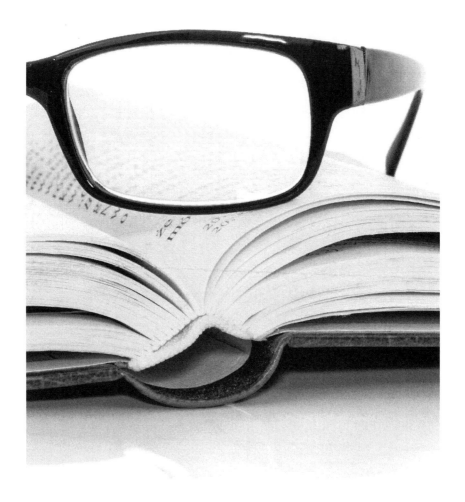

CHAPTER 1
The End of the Story

"...I SMILED AS I left my windows open to let the breeze in. It was a long day. It was also a great day."

I finished the last lines of the book. It put a smile on my face as I thought about the trip that the writer took. There is something about a book that takes you away from your day, but you never leave your chair. A writer has a big job when it comes to carrying all of the readers to a new place and time.

I stood up to stretch. My body had a few aches because I was sitting for over an hour. My brain may have gone on a trip in those pages, but my body did not move. So I took a walk around the room.

I passed the window and looked outside. It was a cloudy day, but there was not a lot of neighbors outside. That meant there was no one to talk to.

I picked up my book off of my reading chair. I walked over to the bookcase and put it back in the place that was just its size. When I looked at all of the books on my shelves, you could tell that I liked to read. I felt like reading again. Reading gave me joy and something new. I wanted that feeling all over again.

I had classic novels. They were thick books, and I did not want to read something that was too long. I had travel books, but I was not planning on a trip anytime soon. Cookbooks were great books, but it was too soon to think about making dinner or even going to the store.

I was getting very disappointed in my book collection. Either I read all of the books or I did not want to start a new book from what I had. I wanted the excitement of a new book.

I walked through my house to the kitchen. Along the way, I passed magazines that I had already read and newspapers that were ready to be recycled.

At that point, I walked outside to see if the mail arrived yet. I was getting bored because I could find nothing to do or read. But when I opened the mailbox, it was empty. I do not know what was worse – a mailbox full of bills or a mailbox that was empty.

"Good morning!" I heard to my left. It was my neighbor Amy. She was a teenager who lived three houses down from mine. She is one of those kids that is too young to drive but old enough to walk everywhere nearby. Today she had a backpack that seemed full and heavy with books.

"Good morning," I answered. "It's Saturday, so why do you have your school books?"

"They are my library books," she said. "I read about one book a day, plus I have some research books I have to return."

"A library book," I said, mostly to myself. "I just finished a book, but I am tired of the ones I have on my shelf."

"Do you have a library card?" Amy asked. "You can find something new at the library for sure."

"I don't know," I said. "It has been a long time since I have gone into a library."

"A long time?" she smiled. "The library has changed since I was a kid. You might be surprised with what you see now."

Amy's smile and the excitement of a new adventure made me curious. I would be bored if I stayed at home. A visit to the library could just be the new and joyful thing I was looking for today.

"How far is the library?" I asked Amy.

"Three blocks," Amy said. "It is on the other side of the city park. And since it is not suppose to rain, you won't need an umbrella."

"May I walk with you?" I asked.

"Let's do it!" Amy said with a smile.

I went back into my house to get my keys and my identification card. Amy said that I had to have a proof of where I lived before I could get a library card. I was looking forward to this visit to the library.

I had never been to the library in town after they built a new one. The old one smelled like musty books and was always too warm. Even the librarians did not seem very nice whenever I went to visit when I was young.

With each step to the library, it felt like I was turning the page of a new adventure book.

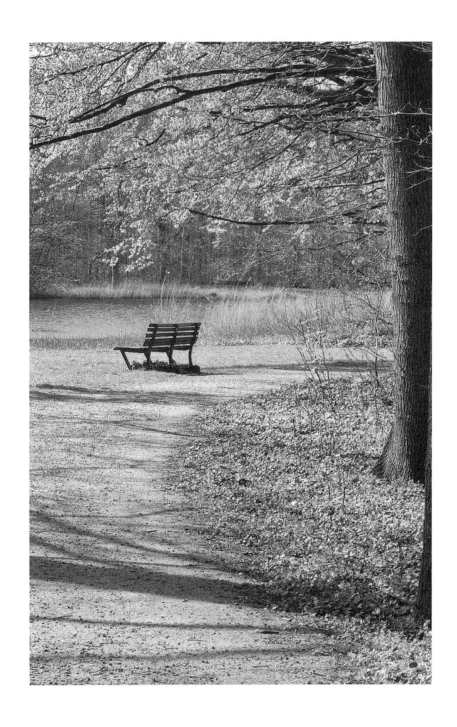

CHAPTER 2
A Walk in the Park

"I LIKE TO READ MYSTERIES," Amy was saying as we walked past the houses on the block. "But I also love fantasy stories. They have monsters, magicians, and things I would never see around my house. Sometimes I like science fiction. Can you believe that there are robots that can do so many things in our life?"

She took a breath. "What kind of books do you like to read?"

"I like stories that are more real," I told Amy. "They have real people doing real things. Sometimes they do things they did not think they could do."

"Like do magic or build a robot?" she asked.

"Not quite," I smiled at Amy. "They learn something for the first time. I just read a book about a sailboat race, so the narrator learned how to sail a boat. Those books are good, but I like travel stories about far-off places."

"Do you travel?" Amy asked.

"I used to," I answered. "I went to six continents, and I loved them all."

"What was your favorite part?" She was getting more interested with each word I said.

"I liked visiting the homes of other people. You can see all of the landmarks like the Tower of London or the Great Wall of China. But you get to really see how people are the same and different when you are a guest in their home."

"Is that why you like nonfiction books, because you like to see what is the same and different to your life?" she asked.

I never thought about it that way, but I think she understood the books I liked to read. "I guess so. But these days I visit people through the stories they write in books."

Amy smiled. "Maybe you should write your own book."

"I have some stories to tell, but I do not have the patience to write them," I told her. "By the time I write the first chapter, my mind is ready for the next story or next adventure. I think I would have an unfinished book every day of the week."

Amy giggled at that idea as she looked both ways at the street crossing. There were no cars on the road, but it was good practice.

The sidewalk went in three directions. Two followed the roads and one went diagonal through the town park. We decided to go through the park because it was quicker.

There was a lot of green grass and park benches along the sidewalk that went through the park. I was too interested in the library to feel like sitting down just yet. Every now and then a runner would pass us. I did not understand why people wanted to run. I was happy with walking.

I could hear birds chirping in the trees above us. If the sun was out, the old trees would give us a lot of shade. There were not a lot of kids playing on the playground either. Amy thought the same.

"My brother is at his soccer practice," she said. "The park is empty because they are at the school fields. He would be swinging as high as he could if he did not have practice."

I remembered playing on the swings at the park. We would swing so high that we would feel the whole swing set shake back and forth.

"The colorful equipment is nice," I said. "We had metal equipment that was hot on sunny days. I think we even had a slide that looked like a rocket, not a tower."

"Cool!" Amy said. "The rocket, I mean. Not the hot metal."

I could see the library at the other side of the park. It was a red brick building that was like many of the other brick buildings in the town. The dark windows kept out the sunlight on brighter days. There were a few cars in the parking lot and about five bicycles at the bike rack. It was built only a few years ago, so it did not have as many old trees around it like the park did.

From the outside it looked like a good place to visit. I thought it had to have thousands of books to choose from. It was so big that I hoped I could find what I was looking for. I had no idea how amazing it would be on the inside.

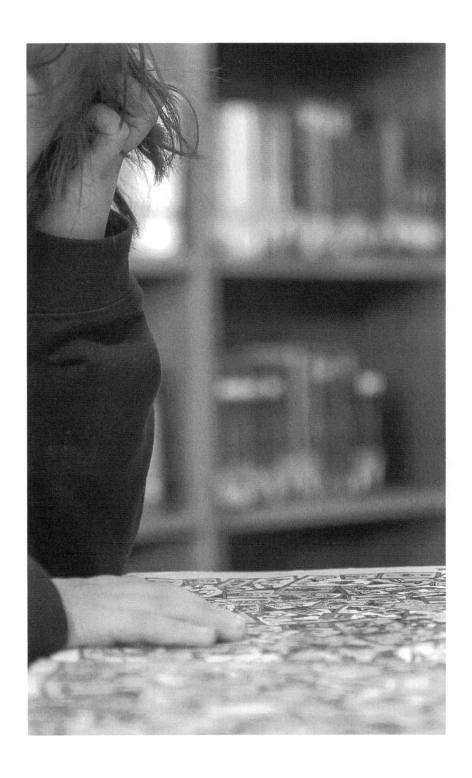

CHAPTER 3
Somewhere Cool

THE FIRST THING that I noticed when I walked in to the library was that it felt cool and comfortable. The second thing that I noticed was the detectors on either side of the entrance. They looked like the posts you see at a store to stop shoplifting. Amy told me that it was way that librarians could tell if items were leaving the library without getting checked out.

The librarian's desk was more like a counter. There was a person who was talking to one of the librarian's standing behind the desk. Whenever she scanned a book, there was a beep to show that it was checked out. That was the only noise that could be heard through the quiet library. At least the only noise from the entrance.

Amy walked to the counter and emptied her backpack. She put books in the slot labeled "book return" and DVDs in the slot labeled "AV return".

"What does 'AV return' mean?" I asked Amy.

"AV means Audio Visual," she said. "That is for movies, CDs, books on tape or CD. There is more than just books here now," Amy smiled.

That was true. After she waved to the librarian, we walked past the librarian's desk and I saw all of the technology the library had. There was a row of desks with computers in each spot. There were racks of recently returned items, and many of them were DVDs.

"The library has a lot of DVDs here," Amy told me. "It is almost like going to a video store, but you do not have to pay for them. Instead you can check them out and return them in a few days for new releases or in two weeks for most DVDs."

That amazed me. I was surprised how much more was in our library. I liked to watch movies, and they had rows of TV shows, travel videos, and even videos for when my grandkids come over to visit.

I must have been thinking of my grandkids because I heard the giggles of children coming from the right of the computer desks. In that wing of the library, there was a section for children.

I remember going to the children's room in my old library that was full of smelly books and a few bean bags. This children's section had tables with puzzles, craft activities, and even some computers of their own as well as many picture books.

"I volunteer during the summer," Amy told me. "They always get helpers from the middle school and high school to work with kids during the summer reading program." She smiled.

"It can be a lot of kids for one librarian, and I get volunteer hours. That will help me when I apply for colleges."

Just like the bright and colorful playground equipment at the park, the decorations of the children's library section was a wonderful way to get kids excited about reading and learning.

I looked at the schedule of events on the door of the children's program room. They had storytime for babies, preschool kids, and even events for teens. I wish they had this when I had kids at home.

"They have programs for adults, too," Amy told me when she saw that I was looking at the children's calendar. We walked back to the computer desks where there were flyers and papers from the library. Among flyers about online safety and lists of resource websites, there was a calendar of events for adults.

The knitting club met here on Monday evenings, board games were played on the third Thursday of the month, and a book club met on the first Wednesday of each month. I was interested in the arts like coloring for adults or painting classes with a local artist.

It was much more than I expected from my library. And we did not even look at the books yet!

Amy moved her empty backpack to her other shoulder. "I need to look for some more books, and the teen fiction is over there." She pointed to a section with taller bookshelves on the other side of the children's section.

"Where are the books," I asked with a grin, "for the older kids?"

"Across from the librarian's desk you will see the doors to the elevator. All of the adult fiction and non-fiction are upstairs."

We agreed to meet at the desk in thirty minutes. I walked to the elevator and tried to prepare myself for what I would see. When the elevator bells went "ding", the doors opened to get me ready for my trip up. It was a quiet trip in the elevator. And when the door opened, I felt like I went to library heaven.

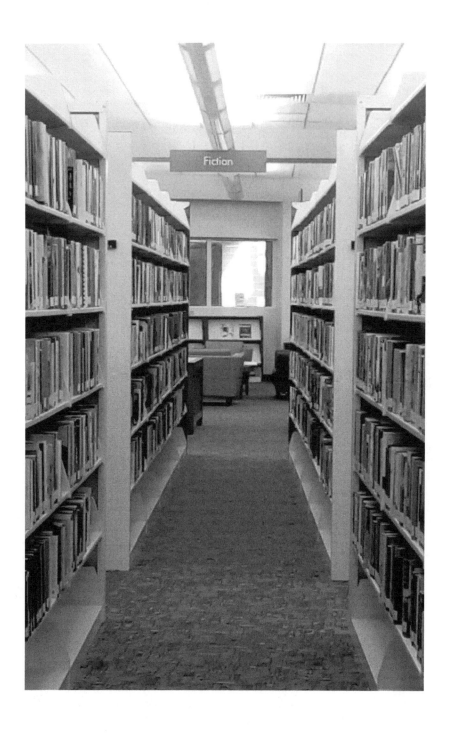

CHAPTER 4
For the Love of Books

I KNEW THE LIBRARY would have many books, but I was amazed by how many books were upstairs.

As I got out of the elevator, I smelled books in a different way. There was a crisp smells of gently used paper from all of the newer books near the elevator.

As I went deeper into the book stacks, there were smells like grass and vanilla coming from the older books in their collection. It was a nice smell that made me feel comfortable and at home.

I was so happy with the collection of books they had. There were rows and rows of biographies, stacks of books about countries far away, and so many books about food. They had cookbooks from famous chefs, all of the different diets, and even the different appliances and cookware for cooking.

I walked around the entire floor so that I could see where everything was. I heard a sound coming from the fiction section and saw a lady come out of the row. She was pushing a cart of books.

"I thought I heard someone come up," she smiled. "Can I help you find something?"

"Right now I am trying to learn where everything is. It is my first time here," I said.

"Well, welcome to your library," she said. "There is a map of our sections over here to help you out," she left her cart by the bookshelves and walked me to the librarian's desk.

"Most of our non-fiction is over here," she pointed, "and here is our fiction section. You will also find large print here," she pointed, "and audiobooks here," she said as she moved her finger across the map.

"Audiobooks?" I asked.

"They are books on CD," she told me. "It used to be that people who had poor eyesight or were blind were the only ones who wanted books on tape. Now when books come out, you can get them on CD read by famous actors or even the author. Many people listen to the books in their car, while they exercise, or just when they are relaxing."

"I like that idea," I said. After the librarian pointed me to the audiobook section, I walked over to see many of the new books and favorite authors.

"Here," she said as she followed me. She handed me a basket, like the ones you see at the grocery store. "Your hands may get full after a while."

I thanked her and chose two books to check out. Then I walked to the large print section. My eyes were still good, but I was curious about large print. I found a book about one of the presidents and found that the large print was so easy to read. I put that book in my basket too.

After I looked at a few more book titles, I went back to the cookbook section. A friend of mine told me about a favorite chef who had many cookbooks. I found a few of those books and decided to try one at home.

The library had so many choices that I was afraid I was going to need a rolling shopping cart instead of a shopping basket for all of the books.

There was a comfy chair near the cookbook section, so I sat down and looked through the cookbooks for a few minutes.

The feeling in that area was calm and peaceful. There was no mean librarian telling people to hush when all they were doing was breathing.

With the children downstairs, it was a quiet place to read, study, and just think. I could see myself coming here just to read when I felt like getting out of the house.

I knew it was almost time to meet Amy, and I still had to get a library card. As I walked back to the elevator, I thanked the librarian who helped me.

"Hope to see you here again soon," she called to me.

I knew that I would be back soon.

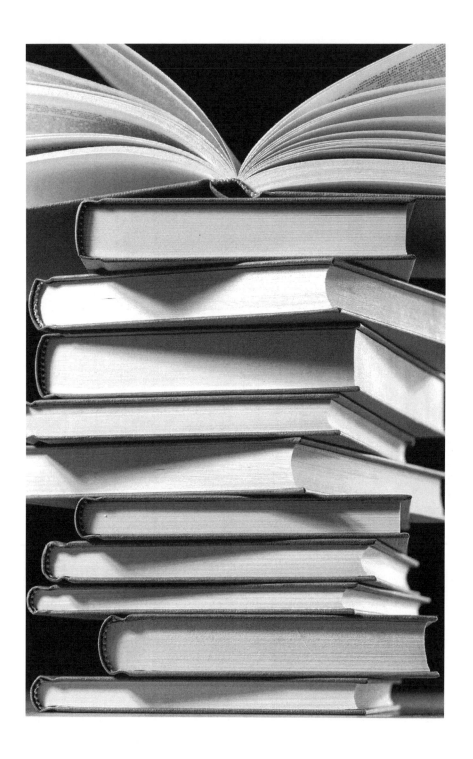

CHAPTER 5
Checking Out

WHEN THE ELEVATOR doors opened on the first floor, there was energy once again. Children were still giggling, a few people were typing on the computers, and the lights just seemed brighter.

I stepped out of the elevator. I saw a rack of books that I did not notice before. It said "Book Sale" on top. I love a good book sale, so I had to see what they had on the shelves.

To my surprise, there were paperback books that were ones I wanted to reread. I loved getting a handful of books for a little money.

It was also nice to know that all of the money from the book sale goes back to the library for new books and materials.

My basket was getting heavy, so I was glad that there was no wait at the librarian's desk. I walked right up and put my basket on the counter.

"Hi," I said. "I would like to sign up for a library card please."

"Wonderful," she said. Her name tag said that her name was Mary. "Do you have your identification with you?"

I pulled my card out of my pocket so that she could put the information in on the computer. It only took a few minutes to fill out forms and sign up. She also asked me to enter a pin number so that I could use the computers any time I wanted.

When I want to sign in on a computer, I just had to put in my library card number and pin for a password.

Just in case that I forgot anything that I could do with my library card, she gave me a pamphlet full of information. I could even check when my books were due back at the library on the website. So much technology!

When my information was ready, she started checking out my books and audiobooks. With each beep, I was excited to know that I had something new to read, new to try, and new to listen to. This was the excitement I was looking for when I finished my book this morning.

"It looks like you found a lot," Amy said as she brought her own bag full of books and DVDs to the counter.

"Some to check out, and some from the book sale," I told her.

"I love the book sale," Amy grinned. "I donated a lot of my books that I no longer read. It helps the library, you know."

I thought about the books on my bookshelf that I knew I would never read again. Maybe it was time for me to donate some of them as well.

After I checked out and paid for my book sale items, I was surprised when Mary put my books in a tote bag. "All new library card holders get a book bag. We hope that you will use it often."

"Oh, I know I will," I said to her.

I waited for Amy to check out as well. She had thick novels, DVD cases, and nonfiction books for one of her assignments.

She told me that many assignments need up-to-date facts from the Internet, but she had a few teachers who wanted to make sure that they knew how to find information in books. She also had to learn how to list it as one of her resources.

The walk back home was better than the walk to the library. The sun was coming out of the clouds. There were children at the playground chasing each other and climbing on all of the equipment.

"Do you know what you are going to read first?" Amy asked me. I told her about the different books I picked out. She agreed with my choice of cookbooks, and she told me about the research project she did on the president from my book.

"Do you ever listen to audiobooks?" I asked Amy.

"No," she said. "I like to hold a book in my hands. Sometimes I may read a book on my tablet, but an electronic book does not have the same feel or smell as a regular book."

When we got to my house, I thanked Amy for inviting me to the library. She thanked me for the company and conversation on our walk. As she walked back to her house, I was in a great mood. The day was getting better and I was happier because of my visit to the library.

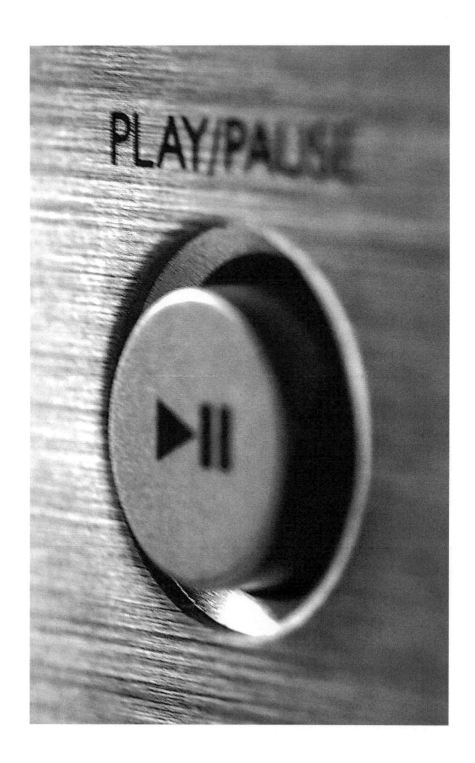

CHAPTER 6
Trying New Things

MY PHONE WAS RINGING when I opened the door to my house. I was able to answer it on the third ring.

"Hello?" I said.

"Hey, it's Michael." My brother also lived in town and we talked to each other every day. "I called you earlier but you were not at home."

"I went to the library today," I said.

"The library? I haven't been there in years," he said.

"Me neither. My neighbor Amy was going and invited me to go with her. Michael, it is nothing like the library when we were kids."

Michael chuckled. "No musty books or mean librarians?"

I laughed with him. "Good-smelling books like in the bookstores and nice librarians. You would like it."

"I drive the new library from time to time," Michael told me. "It looks big."

"And it is not just books," I said. "They have computers, DVDs, and so much more. I bet your grandkids go to some of those children's programs."

"You know, they were telling me how they went to some kind of event about one of their favorite book characters. They were pretty excited about it, too."

"And you are always looking for someone to play chess with you," I said. "They have an event for people to come to just play board games." I giggled. "You could find some new competition who could actually beat you in your own game."

"Now that IS interesting," Michael said. Even though we were on the phone, I could tell that he was seriously thinking about it.

He would like to meet people who knew more about playing games than people in his family. I knew I could never beat him at his own game. "Did you get any books?" he asked.

"I got my library card, then I checked out some biographies and cookbooks. Oh, and I even got an audiobook," I added.

"You mean like books on tape?" he asked. "I know some people who listen to books like that. It sounds a little boring to me, but storytime always did put me to sleep."

"I'll let you know how it goes," I told him.

"Ok, I'll talk to you later then," he said. Then we hung up the phone.

I was ready for lunch, so I went into the kitchen. I already had soup ready to go. As I ate my soup, I looked through the cookbook I checked out. When I found a recipe I wanted to try, I used a small piece of paper like a bookmark to find that page again later.

After I put my soup bowl away, I started a list of ingredients so that I could get them at the store later.

I took a grocery bag from my kitchen and took it with me to my bookshelves. I had to make space for the books that I bought from the book sale.

It felt good to take the books that did not bring me joy anymore and give them a new home. Once I made some space, I put those books that were new to me on my shelf.

By the time I was done, I was ready to relax. Shopping could wait, and I had nothing else planned for the day. I was also excited to start a new book.

I picked up my new book bag from the library and looked at the books I checked out. This may be something I would do once a week or even every few days. No matter what, I knew I could always find something new that could make me happy at the library.

Thinking about new things, I took one of the audiobooks out of my book bag. I read the description again.

It was a book from an author I liked, but it was not one that I read before. The author was the one who was reading it out loud. I never heard their voice before, so I was interested to hear how they sounded. I could imagine that they would put a lot of expression and voices in the characters they made up.

I carefully put the CD into the music player and sat in my reading chair. The author's voice was pleasant and nice to listen to.

While I did not fall asleep during storytime, as Michael called it, I was comfortable as I tried something new.

This gave me more good reasons to enjoy more visits to the library.

Made in the USA
Monee, IL
24 June 2021

72048831R00030